Breastfeeding
TWINS,
Triplets, and
Quadruplets:

195 PRACTICAL HINTS
FOR SUCCESS

Edited by:
Donald M. Keith, M.B.A.
Sheryl McInnes
Louis G. Keith, M.D.

THE CENTER FOR STUDY
OF MULTIPLE BIRTH
In Cooperation With
PARENTS OF MULTIPLE BIRTHS ASSOCIATIONS
CANADA

The Center for Study of Multiple Birth

Suite 463-5
333 East Superior Street
Chicago, Illinois 60611
(312) 266-9093

Cable: TWINSTUDY, Chicago, Illinois, USA

First Published in the United States in 1982
Published simultaneously in Canada

Photographs by Kathryn McLaughlin Abbe and Frances McLaughlin Gill. Cover by Larry Workman. Art by W. F. McWilliam.

Breastfeeding twins, triplets, and quadruplets.
    Bibliography: p.
    Includes index.
    1. Breastfeeding. 2. Twins.
3. Triplets. 4. Quadruplets. I. Keith, Donald M. II. McInnes, Sheryl. III. Keith Louis G.
RJ216.B78   649!3   82-4317

ISBN 0-932254-02-0   AACR2

1st Printing, November 1982
2nd Printing, February 1985

PRINTED IN THE UNITED STATES OF AMERICA

ACKNOWLEDGMENTS

I would like to thank the more than 300 mothers across Canada who provided the information you are about to read. I am grateful for the preliminary work done by Ann Cote, Jan Restall, and Maria Roelofs of the Winnipeg Parents of Twins and Triplets Organization. A very special thanks to Joan Craig, R.N., Kelowna Parents of Multiple Births; M. Levasseur, R.N., Victoria Parents of Twins and Triplets Association; and Linda Pratt, Regina Parents of Twins and Triplets Club for their invaluable help. As mothers who successfully breastfed their twins, they offered much expertise. Chapter 6 "Problems in Breastfeeding and Suggested Solutions," was made possible in part by Julie Tolentino, R.N., and the staff of Parents and Infant Resource Services (P.A.I.R.S.) of Toronto, and members of local chapters of the La Leche League.

This book could not have been written without the foresight of Donald Keith, Executive Director of the Center for Study of Multiple Birth. His patience over the past two years was endless as was the tolerance of my husband and children who helped by taking on household tasks when necessary.

It is also necessary to thank the mothers of twins, triplets, and quadruplets in the United States, Australia, and England who contributed their experiences and offered words of encouragement for this book.

S. McInnes
Executive Assistant
POMBA, Canada

DEDICATIONS

To Jennette Keith, who mothered and breastfed us, with all our love.

Donald and Louis Keith

To the National Organization of Mothers of Twins Clubs, Inc., for their support and encouragement.

Donald Keith
Executive Director

INTRODUCTION

The birth of twins, triplets, or quad-ruplets is a momentous occasion. The pleasure and challenges of parenthood are truly multiplied from the moment you hear that more than one baby is ex-pected. Breastfeeding can be a very joy-ous experience. It brings you and your babies into a close bond of love. How wonderful, then, that these two experi-ences of motherhood can be combined!

The Canadian Pediatric Society and the Canadian Department of Health and Welfare encourage breastfeeding as THE method of choice for infant feeding in Canada. An increasing number of modern mothers share this goal. Many mothers of twins and higher order multiples also desire to breastfeed.

"Breastfeeding Twins, Triplets, and Quadruplets," is a practical guide for women who wish to simultaneously breastfeed two, three, or four infants. Twins are referred to in the general por-tions of this book, but what is said also applies to triplets and quadruplets. The chapter on "Breastfeeding Triplets and Quadruplets" (supertwins) as well as the section "A Note for Mothers of Quadrup-lets" point out differences and special areas of concern.

It is important to recognize that caring for and breastfeeding more than one child at a time places extra demands on the mother's body. It may take time to build up a supply of milk to meet the demands of more than one baby. A sincere desire to succeed, along with a common sense approach in choosing the methods that are best for you, can make this goal attainable. You will need the support of your husband and your doctor.

"Breastfeeding Twins, Triplets, and Quadruplets" will not rewrite the many good books available about the subject of breastfeeding. It supplements this knowledge with specialized information not available elsewhere. Please use the reading and reference guide at the back of this book for additional general information.

"Breastfeeding Twins, Triplets, and Quadruplets" is based on the experiences of mothers who have breastfed their multiples. Methods and alternative suggestions have been collected over a period of years by the Parents of Multiple Births Associations of Canada through questionnaires and personal interviews.

"He" has been used throughout the book to refer to both males and females. It is not our intention to show insensitivity but merely to make the reading easier.

The Editors

CONTENTS

1

WHY BREASTFEED?

General Information

Despite the ever-increasing amount of literature that promotes breastfeeding, and although health agencies and the medical community endorse the practice, there remains some resistance to the idea of a mother breastfeeding twins. A sound knowledge of the methods of breastfeeding and of the many advantages for you and your babies will help you "tune out" those who try to discourage you. Discuss your feelings about breastfeeding with your family. Consult other mothers who have breastfed twins. You can contact them through a chapter of your local Parents/ Mothers of Twins Club or the La Leche League. Your body is preparing for breastfeeding as your pregnancy progresses. Therefore, your decision does not have to be made a long time in advance.

Remember, the size of your breasts is determined by the amount of fatty tissue in them. You can produce milk and breastfeed twins whether your breasts are large or small.

Advantages for Your Babies

- Babies who are breastfed are generally healthier. This is an important consideration if your twins are premature and have a low resistance to infection.

- Breast milk is very easy for babies to digest. Therefore, your twins will probably not be colicky and will almost never be constipated.

- Your babies will not be allergic to your milk and will ultimately be less allergic to other substances. This fact is an important consideration if there is a history of allergies in your family.

- Breastfed babies seldom get fat.

- Breastfeeding is more than a method of feeding. It is a time of close contact between you and your baby and provides the feel of warm skin and the eye contact so necessary for the bonding relationship between mother and child.

Advantages for You

- Breastfeeding is much cheaper than buying bottles and formula for two infants.

- Your body gets back in shape faster
  because breastfeeding causes the
  womb to shrink more quickly.

- Traveling with your twins is easier
  because less equipment is needed.
  In addition, you will not need to refrigerate or warm bottles.

- Breastfeeding can provide you with
  several short, quiet, relaxed periods
  each day. You will appreciate this
  opportunity to sit down and put your
  feet up.

- These relaxed periods allow you to
  get to know each baby. Many
  mothers of twins say that each
  individual baby is not appreciated in
  the blur of necessary activities.

Is the Breast Always Best?

There are some disadvantages to
breastfeeding twins, depending upon your
family situation and the attitude of your
husband:

- You will be feeding frequently for
  several weeks or months. This activity does not go hand-in-hand
  with meticulous housekeeping or a
  busy social life.

- It may be financially necessary for
  you to return to work. Without

special work arrangements, breastfeeding may be difficult.

- Your husband may object to your
breastfeeding. Your marital relationship must be considered along
with the advantages of breastfeeding.

- The circumstances of the birth of
your babies may be such that they
require more nourishment than your
milk can provide in the first few
weeks. If your doctor has
supported your wish to breastfeed
and now is opposed to it, he will
have good reasons. Ask for
explanations and respect your
doctor's wishes. You may
compromise by using your milk as a
supplement to other forms of
nourishment.

- If it is necessary to send one or
both babies to a hospital a distance
from your home, you may have to
reconsider your decision to breastfeed.

The Bottle vs. the Breast

During the past fifty years or so,
bottle feeding and breastfeeding have
been the subjects of some controversy in
medical literature as well as in the
media. Each method of feeding has been

viewed in its own time as a "current fad." At the moment you might be asked, "Why are you breastfeeding?" Seldom, however, will anyone ask your reasons for bottle feeding.

Mothers of twins usually give one answer when asked why they did not breastfeed. They say," I did not have the time." Take a look at this "time" factor. If you breastfeed even ten to twelve times a day, the actual time involved in feeding will be five to seven hours a day. This does not count the changing of diapers, the inevitable spitting up, or the unexpected bowel movements in the middle of a feeding. These inconveniences happen regardless of the feeding method.

In a 24-hour period of bottle feeding, you will spend the same five to seven hours actually feeding your twins. In addition, however, you must add another hour for warming bottles for all feedings and two more hours for washing and sterilizing bottles and preparing the formula. A minimum of three extra hours is needed each day to bottle feed your twins. This time could be spent resting or on other activities.

As the months pass, you will spend less time breastfeeding. The hours spent bottle feeding will also decrease, but you still must take time to prepare all those bottles.

In today's economy, cost must be a consideration in most decisions. Fortunately, nature is on the side of the consumer. The cost to purchase nursing pads, breast pumps, shields, etc., can never begin to equal the cost of bottles, nipples, soap, water, formula, and a sterilizer.

The time factor, along with the high cost of bottle feeding, makes breastfeeding twins the method of choice for many people.

2

PREPARING TO BREASTFEED TWINS

General Information

A good way to start your preparation for breastfeeding twins is to select and read one or more of the in-depth books on breastfeeding from the reading list at the back of this book. This will give you a broad understanding of the process of lactation and the changes you can expect in your breasts during pregnancy and the postdelivery period.

You must know how your body produces milk. Understand and remember the basic rule: "demand will increase supply." This knowledge will help you cope with those first hectic days with two infants. You will be nursing your twins at least seven to twelve times a day, so do not anticipate a rigid schedule of four-hour feedings.

You will spend a good deal of time preparing yourself and your home to receive two or more infants. These changes and related "twin" problems will be covered in Chapter 9, "The Mother of Multiples and Her Family."

Once you have made the decision to breastfeed your babies, discuss your feelings with your doctor. It is essential that he respects your wishes and is prepared to help you with arrangements for breastfeeding if the babies are premature or if you require a Caesarean birth. You should also make an appointment with the pediatrician who will care for the babies after delivery, for it is critical that he supports and encourages your desire to breastfeed your twins.

A part of your preparation for the birth of twins and for breastfeeding is an adequate diet. What you eat must nourish your body as well as the bodies of your infants. Therefore, you will have to increase your food intake with special emphasis on increased protein. You will be eating approximately twice as much as you did before your pregnancy. This, however, does not mean twice as much junk food! Consult your doctor about a proper diet and be very wary of one who sets absolute limits on weight gain. Pregnancy is not the time to diet.

In the later stages of your pregnancy, it may be necessary to eat several small meals during the day in order to avoid the discomfort of three large meals. High protein snacks like cheese and unsalted nuts are good to have on hand. Establish the habit of drinking several glasses of milk or other

liquids with and between meals. Increasing your intake of coffee or tea is not a
good idea.

Although breastfeeding is "natural,"
and the ability to root for the breast and
suck is instinctive for your babies, you
may lack experience and confidence. If
you are a first-time mother, there is no
mechanism for advance training and
practice. Speaking with other mothers
who have breastfed (and, if possible, ob-
serving them while nursing) is about as
close as you can get to that kind of
"hands on" preparation.

Choosing a good brassiere is also a
valuable part of preparation for breastfeeding. Physically preparing your
breasts for the task that lies ahead is
essential.

Suggestions

- Get answers to all of your questions
  both from the doctor who will deliver your babies and from the pediatrician or family practitioner who
  will care for them.

- Determine whether or not both doc-
  tors encourage breastfeeding and, in
  particular, the breastfeeding of
  twins or triplets.

- Make sure your health will continue
  to support your decision even if the

babies come early, are small, or you
require a Caesarean.

- Find out if the hospital where you
will deliver your babies will respect
your wishes that they not be fed
supplements or water between feedings. Since your infants may need to
be placed in the hospital's premature
nursery, ask if you will be allowed to
go in to nurse or have your milk
brought to them.

- Try to locate a milk bank in your
city or find another resource for
"mother's milk" if you are unable to
provide enough when you first begin
to nurse.

- Express your desire, if the delivery
is normal and the babies are of sufficient size, to immediately put
them on the breast.

- See if there is an electric breast
pump available at the hospital or if
one can be rented if required. The
pump may be needed if only one
baby can nurse at first or if both are
too small to be brought to you.

- Use cotton bras because synthetic
materials do not "breathe." The
latter tend to hold moisture in the
nipple area, which may cause the
skin to break down and predispose
the nipples to soreness.

- Avoid bras with plastic or wire supports. They may cause pressure sores, interfere with blood flow as your breasts enlarge, or cause the plugging of a milk duct.

- Purchase a bra with adjustable straps to allow for the increasing weight of your breasts.

- Choose your nursing bra late in your pregnancy. Do not rely on the marked size. Try it on, making sure you can comfortably insert a finger between the material and your skin to allow for swelling when your milk starts to come in.

- Prepare your breasts ahead of time (i.e., toughen the skin of the nipples and encourage the nipples to project if they tend to be flat). Do this in a simple daily routine.

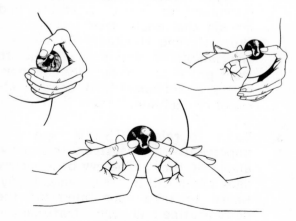

Nipple Protrusion Exercises

- Take your bra off for several hours each day. Wear a soft cotton blouse or T-shirt. If you need the support a bra provides, cut the ends off the cups about an inch back and stitch around the opening. You will get the required support while you expose your nipples to the air, and the constant rubbing against your clothing will toughen the skin. Be sure that this opening does not become too tight as your breasts enlarge.

- Stimulate your nipples by rubbing them gently with a washcloth or towel during your daily bath or shower. Do not use any bath preparations or soaps that contain alcohol or perfume as they will dry and irritate the nipple area.

- Massage hydrous lanolin (from your pharmacy) or cocoa butter into and around the nipple area to keep the skin soft and flexible. Do not use the lanolin if you are allergic to wool products. Avoid any commercial skin softeners that contain alcohol or perfume.

- Learn to relax. This is especially important. Practice relaxation ahead of time. The cry of a hungry baby often will interrupt an activity. Learn to take your mind off the daily routine and concentrate on the needs of your babies. Sit or lie down at various times during the day to clear your mind and relax your muscles. A good way to tune out what is going on around you is to repeat two words to yourself. As you inhale, say "peace" and as you exhale say "tranquil." If you are really tense, tightening your whole body and relaxing groups of muscles from toes to head often works wonders. For some, simply concentrating on even breathing relaxes their bodies.

3

COLLECTING AND STORING YOUR MILK

General Information

In the chapters that follow, we will discuss the actual breastfeeding of your twins. The expressing, pumping, and storage of your milk may be a very important part of your breastfeeding routine.

Hand Expression

Suggestions

● Avoid hand expression before the babies are born. This stimulation of your breasts may release hormones that will cause your uterus to contract.

● Learn how to hand express during the first feeding times after the delivery of your twins. While one baby is at the breast, hand express a little milk from the other breast. One twin's nursing triggers your milk flow. If you try to hand express from breasts that are recently emptied, you will be very discouraged.

• Begin the hand expression with a breast massage. Stroke the breast firmly but gently with the palm of your hand. Move from your chest forward to the nipple area. This massage will probably not be necessary as your "letdown" action becomes established.

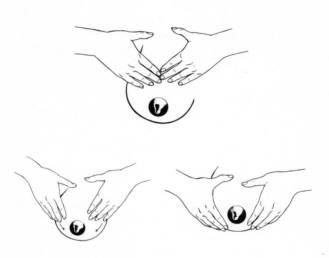

Breast Massage Helps Hand Expression

• Place your thumb and index finger about one inch back from the nipple on the areola, the dark skin around the nipple, after the massage. Press inward toward your chest wall and squeeze gently with your thumb and finger. Remember, first push back and then squeeze.

- Move your thumb and finger to another position around the areola and repeat after you get a drop or two from the first position.

- Sterilize anything that will come in contact with your milk, ALWAYS! Place the bottles or jars you will be using for storage in a saucepan with about two inches of water, cover, and bring to a rapid boil. Shut off the heat, use the lid to drain the water, and leave bottles in the covered pan until needed.

- Collect milk in a sterile bottle or jar, put a lid on it, and refrigerate immediately. You can store your milk in the refrigerator for 24 hours.

- Freeze your milk if you are collecting it for a prolonged period. The milk will be good for about two weeks in a refrigerator's freezer; in the storage freezer, it will last for months. Collect your hand-expressed milk an ounce at a time in a sterile container, chill it, and add it to the frozen supply. ALWAYS leave at least one inch at the top of a bottle in the freezer to allow for expansion. Otherwise, the bottle may burst.

- Do not defrost or slowly thaw the frozen milk before using it. Remove it from the freezer and run the bottle under cold and then warm

water until it starts to liquify. Then
bring the milk to room temperature
in a pan of warm water. Do not remove the milk from the sterile
bottle to warm it.

- Store the amount needed for each
baby for a feeding in a baby bottle
in the freezer for times when you
will be away. If you use disposable
nurser bags, remember to leave
space at the top of the bag to allow
for expansion. Since they are not
made for freezing, such bags often
break open or leak.

- REMEMBER, your milk may appear
watery and bluish and may separate
when stored. Mother's milk does not
look like cow's milk.

The Manual Pump

The manual pump with the rubber
bulb is no longer recommended.
Contamination of the milk may occur if
it runs into the bulb, which cannot be
sterilized. Instead, look for the Evenflo
pump, the Loyd-B-Pump, or the Kaneson
Expressing and Feeding Bottle at your
drug store or where baby products are
sold.

The Electric Pump

General Information

You may need to use an electric pump if (1) you are pumping and storing milk for a newborn baby who has been kept in the hospital, (2) if both twins must remain in the hospital, or (3) a nursing baby is hospitalized and you wish to maintain your milk supply.

Suggestions

- Inquire about the rental of an electric pump at your hospital, medical supply store, or drug store. The local Parents/Mothers of Twins Club or chapter of La Leche League International may be able to help.

- Sterilize all parts of the pump that will be in contact with your milk. ALWAYS!

- Follow <u>exactly</u> the instructions given with a pump.

- Stop using an electric pump if you have a very sore or cracked nipple.

- Do not become discouraged if you can express or pump only a small amount at any one time. Use the collecting and storing methods we have described and the stored milk supply will increase quickly.

- Do not continue pumping after milk stops dripping from the breast to prevent injury to the nipple or breast.

4

BREASTFEEDING TWINS— GETTING OFF TO A GOOD START

General Information

Your breasts produce milk according to the rule of supply and demand. Frequent stimulation, sucking, and emptying of the breasts from the moment of the twins' birth is essential for a good beginning.

During the first week or so, you may experience either nipple soreness at the beginning of a feeding, a sharp pain in the breast as the baby begins to suck, or cramps in the lower abdomen as the uterus contracts. This discomfort is quite normal and will diminish as your breastfeeding routine becomes established. If you are very uncomfortable, ask your doctor about a very mild pain killer.

It is also quite normal to try various positions for feeding the babies either simultaneously or individually. Newborn babies can be very uncooperative when it comes to connecting their mouths with your breast. Many new mothers often feel frustrated trying to find a comfortable position for their own bodies while removing a tiny fist from a baby's mouth or trying to quiet a screamer long enough to give him what he wants. With twins, it seems you just get the knack of breastfeeding one baby when you must start over again with another baby and a different personality. A sense of humor and confidence will see you through these early days.

The amount of time your baby should be on the breast will vary according to hospital "rules." However, the real determining factors are your comfort and the satisfaction of your baby. It may be that you can tolerate only one minute on each breast the first day for each feeding time. Some mothers, though, are comfortable with five minutes or more right from the beginning. Should soreness be a problem, more frequent but shorter nursing times may help.

If you are hand expressing, you may get only a few drops while the breasts are producing colostrum (a yellowish fluid), and only an ounce or less with your first milk. Some mothers who find they cannot hand express very well use either a manual breast pump or an electric pump to stimulate milk production. The essential point is to stimulate both breasts by whatever means possible, at least eight to ten times a day, starting within the first 24 hours after your twins are born.

- Put the babies on the breast immediately if they are of sufficient size and the delivery went well. Within 24 hours after birth, you should be breastfeeding each baby at least eight times a day. In the beginning, your breasts will produce colostrum, which within about three days will be replaced by the "true" milk.

- Insist that both babies be brought to you for each feeding and that you begin night feedings right away.

- Remind the staff that you do not want the babies to receive supplementary bottles of formula or water between feeding times.

- Breastfeed as often as you wish if you are able to have the babies "room in" with you. Your goal is to establish a good milk supply. Therefore, even the sleepy baby should be awakened and fed at least every three hours.

- Begin a regular routine of pumping or hand expressing your milk on the first day if both babies are small and must be kept in the premature or intensive care nursery. This activity should be done ten or twelve times a day. Collect the milk in sterile containers and give it immediately to the nursery staff for refrigeration.

Your milk can then be fed to your babies. It is the best nourishment for them if they are premature. (See Chapter 3, "Collecting and Storing Your Milk.")

- Pump or hand express milk from one breast for a baby who is in a special nursery. Nurse the other baby on the alternate breast. Again, the milk you collect should be given to the nursery staff to feed your other baby.

Breastfeeding After a Caesarean

General Information

A Caesarean delivery need not prevent a good start in breastfeeding your twins. If you have had a general anesthetic, the babies can be brought to you as soon as you are able to stay awake and alert for at least fifteen minutes at a time. Initially, a nurse should remain with you. The procedure is essentially the same after a spinal anesthetic, but breastfeeding times can be more frequent and of longer duration. Further, if you have had an epidural anesthetic, you can probably sit up and breastfeed quite comfortably. Actual nursing time will be short in the beginning but will provide that needed early stimulation. As you become more alert, the nursing can become more frequent and you can hand express or pump between feedings.

Once you are able to breastfeed comfortably on your own, you may find it is easier to breastfeed the babies individually until the soreness from your incision has gone. If you do wish to feed simultaneously, the "football hold" is the best position until this tenderness is gone. (See the section on "Positioning," in this chapter.)

Suggestions

● Have the nurse help you roll onto your side. Place the baby beside you and nurse from the breast closest to the bed. When he is finished, prop the second baby on pillows to reach the other breast.

● Ask the nursing staff for help with expressing and collecting your milk for your babies as soon as possible if your twins cannot be brought to you. Keep in mind the need for early and frequent stimulation of your breasts to build your milk supply.

Home From the Hospital

General Information

It is possible that one or both of your twins will remain in the hospital after you are discharged. This is not an easy situation for you or your family. You may find it beneficial to contact your local Parents/Mothers of Twins Club or a chapter of the La Leche League to talk to other mothers who have successfully "survived" this period of disruption. The important thing is that you continue to maintain a positive attitude and remain confident that soon all of you will be together. By maintaining your milk supply, expressing it, and delivering it to the baby or babies in the hospital, you are giving them the best possible start.

Suggestions

* Maintain the seven to twelve feedings each day for the baby who comes home with you.

* Pump or express milk at each feeding for the baby in the hospital.

* Keep up a schedule of pumping your breasts seven to twelve times a day if both babies remain in the hospital in order to maintain and build the supply until they are able to come home.

* Ask the nurses to instruct you in the proper handling, storage, and transport of your milk if a baby or babies remain in the hospital. Combine the delivery of your milk to the hospital

with an actual nursing of your babies. Do this as often as you can visit the hospital, especially if the babies are not in incubators or if they can be removed from the incubator for short periods.

- Start to establish a good breastfeeding routine in the hospital with co-operation from the nursery staff. There may be a slight interruption in this routine when you come home for you will have increased demands on your time and the babies must adjust to their new surroundings. Your milk may temporarily appear to decrease in volume while the babies may be fussy and hard to settle. Stay calm, rest, and nurse frequently.

- Begin afresh once you and the babies are settled at home if you do not feel you got off to a good start in the hospital. This is an understandable situation with twins. If starting fresh means round-the-clock feedings for a week or so, it will be time well spent in getting to know your babies and in nourishing them. Most women have sufficient milk in seven to ten days to satisfy both babies at a single feeding and the babies should start sleeping at least three hours between feedings.

- Do not allow the clock to rule. You will continue to breastfeed seven to

twelve times a day for several
months if:

- you totally breastfeed without
  supplements

- your twins were very tiny or
  premature.

● Remember that the amount of milk
  you produce depends on the amount
  of stimulation and demand your
  breasts receive from your babies.
  The more frequently you feed them,
  the more milk you will produce for
  them.

Positioning the Twins for Breastfeeding

General Information

There is no one "best way" to
breastfeed your twins. Your comfort and
the ease with which you handle the babies are the determining factors. You
may wish to breastfeed your twins on
demand, separately or simultaneously.
Each method will be covered later.
Many mothers find it difficult to position
tiny babies at both breasts at the same
time without someone to help. Therefore, they only use these positions for
night and early morning feedings when
assistance is available.

- Sit in a large chair with supporting arms, on a sofa with a stool for your feet, or on a bed.

- Use large bed pillows to support your back, other pillows beside your body to support your arms, and still more cushions on your lap to hold the babies at the desired height. Finally, use pillows under your knees if you are feeling strain on your back.

- You can make extra pillows by rolling large towels and putting them in pillow cases. Secure everything with string or rubber bands.

- Experiment with the pillows and the positions we describe since you will have to be comfortable for at least twenty minutes.

Individual Feedings

General Information

Many mothers prefer to breastfeed their twins one at a time to give each baby undivided attention. Some mothers find positions for simultaneous feeding difficult to achieve and become discouraged and tense. In turn, the rewards of breastfeeding are diminished, retarding the letdown of their milk. Spend some time practicing the positions for simultaneous feedings so you can use one if necessary.

The most common procedure for the individual feeding of each baby is to nurse the baby who awakens first. Resettle him when he is finished and then wake the second twin for his feeding. Twins often will adapt to this routine and in a few weeks you may have twenty to thirty uninterrupted minutes with the first baby before the second one cries.

You may find that the breast not being nursed will leak milk in response to the stimulation on the other breast. This leakage should not be significant. To stop it, place the palm of your free hand against the nipple and press firmly for a few seconds. You may wish to collect this leakage in a sterile "scalded" cup or bottle each time and store it in your freezer.

There will be occasions when both twins awaken simultaneously for their feeding even though they normally feed alone. Here are some hints on how to deal with the situation.

Suggestions

- Feed them in one of the simultaneous positions.

- Use a pacifier (soother) for one baby.

30 ● Place one baby in an automatic swing, carriage, stroller, or infant seat, rocking gently with one hand or your foot.

● Use milk previously expressed between feedings that has been stored in a sterile bottle and refrigerated. Warm it and have a helper feed the second baby while you breastfeed the first baby. Even a little milk will help satisfy him. You can then place him at the breast to finish feeding after the first baby is finished.

● Feed your babies in quick rotation. Sit on a bed or sofa with your back supported by pillows. Place a twin on each side of you with a pillow on the other side of each child to prevent a sudden roll. Use a pacifier to soothe and calm one baby while you pick up and breastfeed the other for about three to five minutes. Burp him if necessary and replace him at your side. Place the second baby at your breast for the next three to five minutes. Repeat this rotation until both babies are satisfied.

Method A "The Crisscross Hold."

General Information

    This is a difficult position to maintain with tiny, weak feeders or with babies who need frequent burping. It becomes much easier after about six weeks when the sucking instinct is stronger and the twins "latch on" securely.

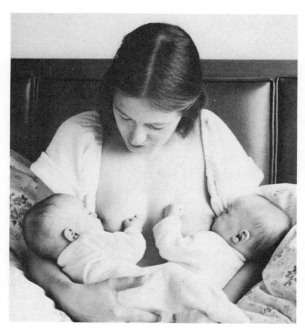

Crisscross Position

- Sit with your back well supported and place a pillow under each elbow and on your lap.

- Place the first baby in the normal nursing position.

- Put the second twin across his twin's body so that they are crisscrossed, facing each other, one at each breast.

- Support their backs with your arms and clasp your hands at their buttocks to pull the babies close to you.

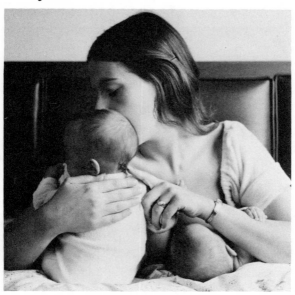

One Position for Burping

- Burp the babies by: (1) sitting both babies forward, crossing your arms to support each chin in your hand, (2) by releasing one twin at a time and sitting him forward, or (3) by pulling each twin up onto your shoulder.

Method B "The Football Hold."

General Information

This position can be used with tiny babies and is easier to achieve without help. You will need several pillows and you should sit on a bed or sofa.

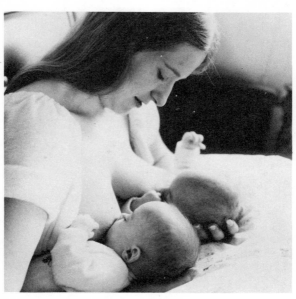

Football Hold

- Place a pillow on each side of you, one lying lengthwise across your lap, and one under your knees to keep them slightly bent in order to prevent back strain.

- Put one baby on each of the pillows at your side. Position them with their feet facing backward and their faces toward your face.

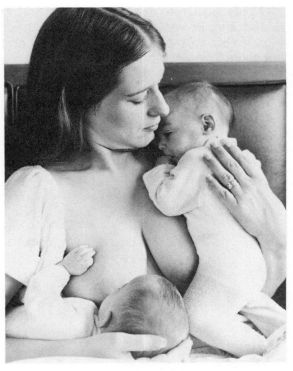

Another Position for Burping

- Pull them forward onto your breasts, with your hands holding each baby's head. Use your arms to hug the babies close to your body.

- Adjust the pillow on your lap as necessary to bring the babies' heads higher than their feet and to keep them rolled slightly on their sides.

- Burp one or both simultaneously by pulling them forward and toward you up onto your shoulder.

Method C "The Parallel Hold."

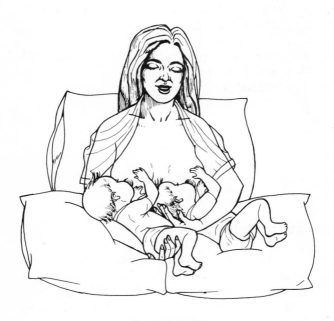

Parallel Hold

This position is a variation of the crisscross hold. Some mothers find it more comfortable.

Suggestions

● Sit with one baby at each breast. Face both babies in the same direction, their bodies parallel. One will be held in the normal nursing position, the other one alongside him with your arm around his body, his head cupped in your hand.

● Use pillows as needed to support their bodies.

● Burp the babies by sitting them forward or pulling them up onto your shoulder.

Method D "Front V Hold."

General Information

This is the best method for night feedings and is very helpful if you cannot sit comfortably right after delivery. Use pillows to support yourself in a half lying position on your back.

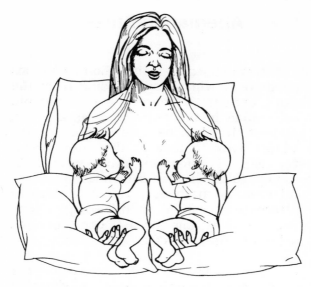

Front "V" Hold

Suggestions

● Place a baby at each breast, facing
the other, with their feet pointing
away from you, their knees meeting
in a "V."

● Support both of their backs with
your arms, your hands cupping their
buttocks, to hold them securely at
your breasts.

● Burp the babies by sitting forward
and bringing them into an upright
position.

Alternating Breasts

Mothers differ in their opinions about one twin always feeding from the same breast. If there is a considerable difference in the twins' size or appetite at first, it might be wise to allow a particular twin to feed at the same breast for each feeding to allow your milk supply to meet the demand. As these differences disappear, you can start to alternate breasts at each feeding or feed one baby at one breast one day and alternate the next day.

For good brain development your twins should receive visual stimulation from both sides. Therefore, alternate breasts or vary the holding position on occasion. Some mothers are concerned that if one baby is a bigger eater and is kept on one breast, the breasts will appear lopsided. This rarely happens.

The Care Chart

Many mothers recommend keeping a "care chart" for all aspects of baby care. Breastfeeding information can be included to help you keep track of which side or position was used at what feeding and how the baby nursed. A sample is shown.

SAMPLE CARE CHART

TIME	STARTING BREAST (LEFT/RIGHT)	POSITION	MINUTES ON BREAST	SUPPLEMENT (YES/NO & AMOUNT)	NUMBER OF WET DIAPERS	BOWEL MOVEMENT	BATH	MEDICINE	VITAMINS	ADDITIONAL NOTES

Supplementing

General Information

Modern parents have become so well acquainted with "schedules" for babies that they automatically assume all babies will hold to the traditional four- or three-hour feedings. Mothers strive, then, to make the babies accommodate to them rather than adjusting to their babies' needs. This thought process may make you feel that your milk is inadequate and that your babies need a supplement. Breast milk is very easily digested by your babies, and they may be hungry every two to three hours. Your breasts accommodate to this need, producing enough milk in one-and-a-half to two hours after a feeding to satisfy that hungry baby. Therefore, it is wrong to assume that your babies need a formula supplement simply because they require frequent feedings.

There is a strong relationship between the amount of formula supplement you use and your milk production. If you come to rely on formula because you are rushed or too tired to breastfeed and do not empty your breasts, less milk is produced for the next feeding. The result, over a period of several days, is the weaning of your babies. Ultimately, you will be faced with the task of trying to breastfeed AND prepare bottles and formula.

You may, of course, be concerned about the amount of milk the babies are receiving when you do not have the reassurance of ounces clearly marked on a bottle. For mothers of tiny twin babies this worry can reach "nightmare" proportions.

Relax! You are supplying enough milk if you are getting six to eight soaking diapers from each baby in a day; if you are feeding seven to twelve times a day; and if the baby has good color, clear eyes, and is alert during waking times. Premature infants can be very slow weight gainers in the first few weeks. It is the constant steady gain that counts—not the actual number of pounds the baby weighs on a given day.

One mother was frantic over what appeared to be a slow weight gain in her twins. At three months, they weighed only nine pounds. She wanted to supplement until the doctor reminded her that the babies were two months premature and weighed only four pounds at birth. The actual gain over three months, then, was more than adequate.

Suggestions

• Think carefully about what starting a supplement will mean before you begin. Ask yourself whether it is your expectations for a "schedule" that makes you think supplementing is required.

- Remember, babies cry for reasons other than hunger. Their need for sucking goes beyond just feeding. Perhaps just holding him for a few minutes with the pacifier is all that is needed for the baby who seems to cry constantly or who settles down for half an hour and then cries again.

- Take a day off. Take the babies to bed and nurse around-the-clock if you feel your milk production is low. You can sleep when they are sleeping or catch up on some reading or mending. Increase your liquid intake at the same time. You will certainly benefit from this rest and it may be all that is needed to increase your milk supply.

- Do not watch the clock! Many mothers make the babies adapt to their needs and think that perhaps a little supplement at the four o'clock feeding will mean they can have supper on time and without interruption.

- Use a supplement of formula or baby cereal mixed with your milk when it is required. Use it when the doctor suggests it (because he is concerned about the babies' weight gain), if you are ill, or if you have a breast infection that requires a limited amount of sucking or expressing of your milk.

- Empty your breasts of as much milk as you can FIRST. Start decreasing the amount of supplement and nurse more frequently to rebuild your milk supply as the situation improves.

Starting Solids

General Information

With twins, there is a temptation to use baby cereals as a means of lengthening the time between feedings, particularly the night feedings. In general, young infants do not digest or absorb the food from this type of feeding. What you are doing is filling stomachs and cutting back on nutrition. You also may be decreasing your milk supply by nursing less frequently. Your doctor will advise you about the need for and time to start feeding solids.

Common Questions and Answers

Will I have to nurse frequently?

It is difficult to generalize because each mother and her babies present a different situation. Many mothers have a lot of milk right from the start and develop an easy routine very quickly. Others must work at establishing a milk supply for two babies. As a rule, you will be nursing seven to twelve times a day for the first six weeks to three months and may have to maintain a minimum of eight nursing times a day until the babies are five or six months old. Ignore the clock and meet your babies' needs! If you have to be away for periods during the day or if you need a break in the evenings, collect as much milk as possible each day so you have a supply for these times.

How do I know the babies are receiving enough?

Each baby is receiving enough milk if:

- you are nursing each baby seven to twelve times in every 24 hours

- each twin is gaining about one pound a month

- you have six to eight soaking diapers per day for each baby (supplemental water throws off your diaper count).

What if one or both of the twins are not gaining enough weight?

Discuss ideas for temporary supplements with your doctor. The aim is to keep them gaining weight while you build up your milk supply to keep them healthy and growing on breast milk alone.

Always breastfeed <u>first</u>, then offer a
supplement if necessary. Since a baby
uses a different sucking method with a
bottle and rubber nipple, he might
become confused. Try using a Nuk orthodontic nipple or giving the supplement
by spoon or eyedropper. If the reason for
the babies not gaining weight appears to
be a low supply of milk, try nursing more
frequently. Remember: the more you
breastfeed, the more milk you will produce.

Should I use a pacifier?

No, not if the pacifier is a replace-
ment for nursing because you are too
busy or too tired and want to postpone a
feeding. It is much easier on you and on
your babies to take the half hour and
feed them than it is to listen to fussy
babies.

Yes, there are times when a pacifier
may be needed and you do not have to
feel guilty about using one. Again, the
best type, in order to avoid nipple confu-
sion, is the Nuk orthodontic pacifier.

How much time should I spend nursing?

The babies probably get the bulk of
your milk in the first five to seven
minutes of each nursing period, but their
need for sucking may go beyond that. A
rule of thumb is fifteen to twenty
minutes for each baby. Babies have different personalities. One of your twins

may be a "gulper"—he takes what he needs and turns away in ten minutes. The other one may be slow and steady and want to remain on the breast for twenty minutes or more. Another factor to be considered is any nipple soreness you may be experiencing. If you cannot tolerate a long period of breastfeeding, you may have to nurse more frequently and for shorter periods until the soreness disappears.

Will I ever establish a routine that I can count on?

Yes, with time and patience your daily baby care and feeding will fall into a routine. Look, however, for:

- days when one or both of your twins will constantly need to be fed. These times usually last only 24 to 48 hours.

- growth spurts, which usually occur at about two weeks, six weeks, three months, and six months. The babies need added nutrition during a time of growth, and this means you must increase the frequency of nursing for a few days. Identical twins are more likely to have growth spurts at the same time while fraternal twins will probably develop at different rates.

Take a good look at what you are eating. Are you thinking more about your waistline than about food intake? You must eat good, balanced, high energy foods. You need high protein foods from the meat, eggs, and cheese groups, along with carbohydrates from the cereal and bread groups; and the vitamins and minerals from fruits and vegetables. You may require a vitamin and mineral supplement, so ask your doctor to recommend the best combination for you.

Check your liquid intake. Is it high enough? If you are totally breastfeeding you need up to three quarts of fluid a day. Make a conscious effort to drink water, milk, and juices with each meal, as you are breastfeeding, when you get up in the morning, and right before bedtime.

Are you getting enough rest? Perhaps you are trying to do too much too soon. Housework will wait, and others can do it for you. Every group of mothers of twins laughingly tells stories about dust balls and unmade beds. Accept the situation as a fact of life for a mother with two infants.

How long should I breastfeed my twins?

That is entirely up to you. Many mothers breastfeed for the first year or more while just as many find that they wish to wean their twins after three months. What you must consider is whether weaning early is going to create more or less work for you. If you wean before your twins are taking solids and can be given a cup for milk, you will be spending those hours handling bottles and formula. Each mother must decide for herself.

How do I handle a baby who seems to reject the breast?

A full-term baby usually has a very strong sucking reflex. However, in the beginning, your baby may show very little interest in feeding and will only stay on the breast for a minute or less at some feeding times. Do not force him or worry about it. As your milk comes in, his interest will increase. If he still seems reluctant, snuggle him close and express a little milk into his mouth. He will soon get the connection between the warm skin contact and the warm milk he receives.

Perhaps he is reluctant because his mouth is not positioned correctly on your breast. After the initial letdown he is working hard and getting nothing. It is necessary for your baby to take the nipple AND the dark skin area, the areola, into his mouth in order to apply sufficient pressure to keep the milk flowing. If an older baby suddenly rejects the breast, it may be because he is teething, has some nasal congestion from a cold, or is uncomfortable in the position in which you are holding him.

He may also be distracted by the activity going on around you. Try a new position at the breast and go into a quiet room for awhile. Offer him the breast the usual number of times a day, let him take what he can or will at each feeding, and feed the other twin more frequently to keep your breasts empty. If this goes on for more than a couple of days, consult your doctor because you may have to offer a supplement for awhile.

Do I have to burp my babies during a feeding?

Because breastfed babies do not take much air into their stomachs as they suck, they often will not require burping until the end of a feeding. If, however, one of the babies has been crying a great deal prior to feeding, he may need several burpings during a feeding. Some babies always need burping and others seldom do. You will soon learn the individual needs of your twins.

How often will the babies have bowel movements?

Breastfed babies who are not receiving other supplements do not get constipated. The "normal" bowel movement for a breastfed baby is very soft, often curdy and unformed, and will range from yellow, to yellow-green, to brown in color. Some babies have a bowel movement after every feeding. Others may go for several days between large bowel movements. A lapse of time between bowel movements does not indicate constipation. Rather, the sign of constipation is hard, dry stools. Each twin may vary a great deal in the size and number of his bowel movements.

Will medications I take affect the babies?

Some medicines you take will pass through to your babies; others will not. If you take routine medications like aspirin for headaches, antihistamines for allergies, or cold remedies that need no prescription, make a list of them and the brand names and ask your doctor if they will affect your babies. If they do, you might consider going without or trying something less strong. When your doctor prescribes medications, always remind him that you are breastfeeding.

5

BREASTFEEDING TRIPLETS AND QUADRUPLETS

General Information

Everything you have read about breastfeeding and, in particular, about breastfeeding twins applies to triplets, and quadruplets—with one exception. That is the possibility of simultaneous feeding of all the babies. Consider some different techniques and alternatives.

First, and above all, you must have confidence in your own ability to breast-feed your babies AND the absolute support of your husband, doctor, and the nursery staff. A daily helper in your home for the first six weeks is almost essential. This may mean sacrifices in other family financial plans. Your doctor, the hospital social worker, or an employment agency can direct you to the type of household or baby-care worker you will need and can afford. With triplets or quadruplets, there is an increased chance that one or more of the babies will be small and remain in the hospital after you are discharged. It is still possible to breastfeed by using the collecting and storing methods described in a previous chapter.

Having three or four babies can contribute to marital tension. As hard as it may be while you are in the midst of this experience, try to put these months into perspective. For both you and your husband, this is a small portion of your total married life. For your babies, however, it is a most important time. The care of your babies will require cooperation and teamwork for many years to come. A beginning filled with humor and patience is essential.

In Canada, the United States, the United Kingdom, and Australia support systems are now available to help you. Within the Parents of Multiple Births Associations (POMBA) in Canada, there is a Parents of Triplets Council, consisting of a network of representatives across the country who are mothers and/or fathers of triplets and quadruplets. They will be happy to answer your questions or to put you in touch with another mother close by. In the United States, the Center for Study of Multiple Birth maintains a "Supertwin Registry." Parents who join will be referred to other parents who can assist with a particular problem or share their experiences with you. The National Organization of Mothers of Twins Clubs, Inc., will refer you to a local chapter which can usually tell you if there are "supertwins" in the area. Similarly, in Great Britain and Australia, the National Associations have recently formed a "Supertwins" branch which also puts parents in touch with other parents in similar circumstances. Addresses for all of these organizations are in the concluding chapter, "The Benefit of Experience."

Some mothers say it is not outright criticism of trying to breastfeed their babies that disturbs them. It is the sly comments and sighs of exasperation from the hospital staff that almost makes them give up breastfeeding. Each mother realizes, however, that this is her own individual decision. Every mother of triplets or quadruplets has the right to try breastfeeding her babies without interference.

You will definitely have enough milk for your infants if you work to build up your milk supply by meeting the demands of your babies and not relying on supplements any longer than is necessary.

Suggestions (from mothers of triplets and quadruplets)

- Breastfeed each baby as often as possible. Total breastfeeding is possible. As you build your milk supply to satisfy the needs of your babies, you may have to use a supplement of formula or expressed milk from another mother for part of each feeding. As the supply of your own milk builds, you can decrease the amount of supplement.

- Increase your food consumption, yet eat wisely. This is essential. Build your fluid intake to a minimum of three quarts (twelve full glasses) every day.

- Use your helper to get the required amount of rest. Do not work with her. Rest while she does the housework and cooking.

- Get off to a good start by having one or all the babies on the breast at least seven times in the first 24 hours after birth. If the babies are not able to leave the nursery, begin hand expressing or pumping immediately and repeat often during each day.

- Be firm with the nursing staff. Make sure the nurses realize that breastfeeding is important to you, and ask them not to give supplements to the babies.

- Be reasonable. Premature babies may require more nutrition than you can supply at first. Ask your doctor to explain his reasons if he insists on supplementing.

- Have the babies brought to you one at a time, at first. Put each one on the breast starting with Baby A on one side for one to five minutes and Baby B on the other side for one to five minutes. Allow Baby C to empty both breasts. Bottle feed Baby D. At the next feeding, start with Baby C and Baby D and repeat this procedure.

- Maintain this rotation once you are at home. Always breastfeed each baby first and then offer a supplementary bottle if they are not satisfied. Reduce or discontinue this supplement as your milk supply builds.

- Consult your doctor and pediatrician about the availability of mother's milk from a milk bank or other source in case it is needed in the early weeks.

- Use a care chart to keep track of this rotation, but do not waste time. Hang a clipboard on each crib and jot notes on it as you settle the baby.

- Use the system best suited to your circumstances. Do not be afraid to experiment and do not be discouraged if one feeding does not go well. Some mothers find that using one of the "twin" positions for two babies followed immediately by the third and fourth is faster and easier. Others have worked out a complicated system of rotation using individual or simultaneous twin feeding positions combined with bottles of their collected milk or formula.

- Obtain encouragement from other mothers who have breastfed more than one baby. Contact your Parents/Mothers of Twins Club and La Leche League chapter as soon as you know you are having triplets or quadruplets and maintain that contact by telephone if getting out to meetings is not possible at first.

A Note for Mothers of Quadruplets

General Information

Mothers of quadruplets have successfully breastfed their babies. Sometimes, through a rotation system, a mother will breastfeed one or two babies while bottle feeding the others. Breastfeeding cannot necessarily be recommended for all mothers of quadruplets. However, if you do have in-home help, the babies are a good weight and can be taken home together or can be fed outside of the incubators, and you and your doctor feel they would benefit from breastfeeding, by all means do try.

Suggestions

- Get off to a good start by breastfeeding at least one of the babies, if possible, and start the routine of pumping and collecting your milk immediately after birth.

- Rotate the babies for breastfeeding and then complete the feeding with the recommended formula.

- Breastfeed two at a time in one of the "twin" positions, completing the feeding with formula.

- Alternate breastfeeding and bottle feeding two babies at each feeding.

- Use daily or live-in help.

- Try to breastfeed for at least the first six weeks to give the babies a good start; most mothers of quadruplets stop nursing after two months.

- Consider the use of milk from a human milk bank.

6

PROBLEMS IN BREASTFEEDING AND SUGGESTED SOLUTIONS

General Information

In the first weeks as a new mother of twins, you undergo many emotional and physical changes. Typically, small annoyances become major problems when sleep is in short supply and when you are feeling unsure of your ability to cope with two infants. Most of the difficulty is related to the "twin situation" rather than to breastfeeding itself. Treat problems as they occur and stay calm. Your best source of information is another mother of twins who has breastfed. She will offer advice that has been tried and works or will let you know if a doctor should be consulted.

Engorgement

General Information

Engorgement is the swelling of the breast tissue that occurs when your milk first comes in or when you have gone a long period between feedings. Many mothers never experience engorgement.

- Nurse your babies as soon as you can after birth and keep feeding them frequently to prevent engorgement.

- Begin hand expression or pumping within the first 24 hours after they are born if you are separated from them by special nursery restrictions. Maintain the stimulation and flow of your milk by expressing seven to twelve times every 24 hours.

- Breastfeed your babies or hand express milk to prevent or alleviate engorgement. Frequent nursing or expression probably will mean you will never experience engorgement. Hand express milk from both breasts at regular intervals if you must be absent for a feeding or series of feedings.

Sore Nipples

General Information

With or without prenatal nipple preparation, you may experience nipple tenderness in one or both breasts. Many mothers of twins experience this discomfort. Some have commented that it was a part of their nursing experience from the beginning until they weaned many months later. Other mothers never had the problem at all. Again, each woman and her babies will have different degrees of discomfort for varying periods of time.

Suggestions

- Do not stop breastfeeding. Soreness is due to tender skin and will only start again once you resume.

- Feed the babies, one at a time, while the pain persists. Start on the unaffected side, then switch to the sore nipple. Start the second baby on the sore side and then switch to the unaffected breast.

- Vary the position for holding your babies so that their mouths are applying pressure all around the nipple and areola.

- Toughen the skin on your nipples by exposing them to the air. Leave the nursing flaps down and wear a blouse that buttons up the front so you can "cover up" when necessary.

- Nurse for shorter periods but more frequently for a few days.

- Never pull a baby away from your breast. Rather, release the suction by inserting your finger between his tongue and your nipple. Also do not allow the baby to "chew" on your

nipple. When he is getting no more
milk and/or his hunger is satisfied,
remove him from the breast.

- Apply a cream or ointment to soothe
  sore nipples.   Pure lanolin works
  very well, and when applied lightly
  does not have to be removed before
  feeding. Your doctor may prescribe
  an ointment. If so, be sure to ask
  whether it needs to be washed off
  before feeding.

- Seek a mild pain reliever from your
  doctor if necessary. Do not self-
  medicate.

Cracked Nipples

General Information

A small crack or fissure may form
on the nipple, the areola, or on the area
where nipple and areola meet. This can
be very painful and should receive
treatment the minute you notice it. Begin the procedures described for a sore
nipple and try the following:

Suggestions

- Keep the nipple dry and exposed to
  the air between feedings.

- Do not remove any scabbing, there-
  by prolonging the healing process.

- Consult your doctor about using an antiseptic cream on the cracked area. It must be washed off before nursing the babies.

- Use a nipple shield for a day or two (but no longer than that), if feeding is very uncomfortable. The shield is a plastic or rubber disc shaped like your breast with a nipple attached. It prevents direct contact of the babies' mouths on your nipple, but it does not allow complete emptying of your breasts. If you must use it for a complete feeding, immediately hand express the breast until it is empty. Prolonged use of the shield may inhibit your milk supply. Try using the shield at the beginning of the feeding just until letdown occurs, after which sucking is not as painful.

- Replace the nipple in a Davol #773 nipple shield with a Nuk orthodontic nipple. The Davol shield is the most effective and the Nuk nipple provides a sucking method closest to actual nursing.

- Express your milk and feed your babies by bottle if you must stop nursing for a day or two. (See "Collecting and Storing Your Milk," Chapter 3.)

- Look for the products mentioned in this book; they are available from stores where baby products are sold or from drug stores. Your local chapter of Parents of Twins, La Leche League International, or Public Health Unit may also direct you to the best source.

Blocked Duct and Breast Infection

General Information

A milk duct becomes blocked because of general engorgement or because of an ill-fitting bra on one area of the breast. This sometimes leads to inadequate emptying from one duct. Your milk then backs up in the sinuses behind the duct and appears as a lump that can get very red and painful. This pressure must be relieved or it may lead to a mastitis (inflammation of the breast) or develop into a breast infection.

Suggestions

● Do not stop breastfeeding; more frequent feedings may clear up a plugged duct very quickly.

● Suspect dry crusts over one area of the nipple. This may indicate that you have a blocked duct. Soak the area with a warm, wet washcloth to remove the crusting.

- Express your milk by hand to make sure the breast is empty after a feeding.

- Get early treatment of a breast infection. THIS IS ESSENTIAL. If you notice a lumpy or hard area in your breast accompanied by a fever or general body ache, you may have an infection. You may not be required to stop nursing from the affected breast. Talk with your doctor; tell him how important you feel it is to maintain your milk supply for your twins. Ask him for a treatment plan that includes alternatives to a complete stop.

- Apply warm, wet compresses; get plenty of rest and hand express while you are waiting to see the doctor. DO NOT feed this milk to your babies until the physician makes a diagnosis.

- Continue feeding from the unaffected breast.

Leaking

General Information

The letdown of your milk may occur at inopportune times. This problem may dissipate as your milk flow becomes established or it may linger throughout your breastfeeding experience.

- Cross your arms and press firmly when you feel the tension prior to the milk flow. This technique is unnoticeable and works for most women.

- Wear breast pads inside your bra. Avoid using the type that have a plastic back. They hold moisture which could result in soreness or cracks in the nipple.

- Prevent the staining of good clothes when you go out by using the plastic-backed type just for these brief periods of time.

- Make inexpensive breast pads. Cut disposable diapers into pieces and remove the plastic backing. Use clean, white hankies that can be laundered. Purchase a small length of white cotton and cut it into squares. Cut up cotton diapers. Avoid the flannel type of diaper because lint may collect and form a crust on the nipples.

7

WEANING

General Information

There is no predetermined age for weaning your twins. Rather, it is either your decision or the babies'. The former is called "mother-led" weaning; the latter, "baby-led" weaning. There are many reasons why you might decide at any time to stop nursing your babies. Be aware, however, that weaning does not cure problems. It will not make a fussy baby settle down or sleep through the night. It will not make you suddenly feel more rested or give you more time for other things. It is up to you to decide how long weaning will take and what feedings you will stop and when.

Some mothers become depressed at the ending of this special time with their twins. View weaning as a positive step in the growth of your babies. Remember that most mothers feel the same way when their children start school, leave home for the first time, or get married. All these experiences are a part of being a mother.

Suggestions

- Start introducing an occasional bottle of your milk by two to three

months if you wish to stop nursing 67
before six to eight months. This
helps ensure that your baby will take
a bottle when the weaning process
starts.

● Do not introduce a bottle by prop-
ping it. Your babies still need to be
cuddled during feeding.

● Consult your doctor about weaning
to prepared formula or cow's milk.

● Watch your babies for reactions to
this substitute of bottle for breast.
Look for a response to the formula
or milk (rash, diarrhea, or constipation). Check if your babies suddenly
are fussier or begin to suck their
thumbs. If either case occurs, it
may be wise to resume breastfeeding for a week or two and then try
again.

● Try substituting bottle for breast at
a rate of about one feeding per day,
each week. Start with the feeding
your babies are least interested in
(or the feeding that is least conve-
nient in your daily routine). Continue this gradual change until you
are nursing only once a day. Often
the early morning or bedtime feeding remains because it is the one
most enjoyed by you and your babies. You may wish to continue inde-
finitely with this particular breastfeeding time each day.

• Let your babies "lead" if you are in no hurry to wean. From about eight to eighteen months, as your twins become more active and more aware of each other, they may forget a feeding. They will be taking solid foods and will start to eat with the family. Finally, they will settle into a three-meals-a-day routine, possibly nursing before naps and bedtime. Start substituting with a bottle or cup as you see this happening. Between eight months and a year you will probably wean to a bottle, as many babies do not get enough milk from a cup. Also remember that many babies need the sucking provided by a bottle well past the first year. After a year of age, they should be able to handle the cup well and get enough liquids from it at meals and snack times. Watch for your babies' reactions.

• Substitute without decreasing your physical contact with your babies. Give juice or milk with the babies on your lap while you read or sing to each baby. Feeding is more than just getting and giving nourishment. All babies need warmth and lots of cuddling.

• Cut down on the liquids you are consuming and eat less while you are weaning. You have established a habit of eating and drinking a great deal and, for some, weaning brings on a weight gain. You may experience a slight fullness in your breasts and some leakage for several weeks after weaning, along with the feeling of "letdown" of milk when your babies cry.

8

PERSONAL CARE

You must learn to take care of yourself while you make adjustments in your household and establish a care and breastfeeding routine for your babies. You will need extra rest, a balanced diet, and time to care for your breasts.

Rest

General Information

It will not be easy to find moments for relaxation. You may think you will never have a full night's sleep again. Remember, as your baby care routine becomes established, there <u>will</u> be times for an extra nap.

Suggestions

- Go to bed after the evening feeding. Relax with a book if you are not sleepy right away.

- Nap during the day when the babies do, whenever possible.

- Take older children who do not nap into the room with you and lie down to read them a story.

70

- Get your feet up when your husband comes home in the evening. This may mean an early supper and bath for your older children.

- Plan simple meals that can be prepared earlier in the day when you are busy in the kitchen. Let your husband put a casserole in the oven or start the vegetables while you relax.

- Ask your husband to take over the after-dinner tasks while you sleep until the evening feedings.

- Accept offers of help. Most mothers find the hours from 5 p.m. to 8 p.m. the hardest to handle. Ask family members or hired help to come at that time. Students can be valuable helpers and are happy to prepare an occasional meal for you. Lie down and rest when help is there.

- Do not use free time to get extra housework done; it will wait. Rest!

- Investigate the possibility of using a homemaker service through your local Red Cross or Community Services Organization.

- Look for information on live-in "nannies." The information is available in Canada at Manpower and Immigration Offices or employment agencies.

- Interrupt your busy routine with a relaxation exercise. Lie on the floor and breathe deeply. Tighten your whole body. Exhale and go limp. If you cannot lie down, take a deep breath, stretch your body, exhale, and let your body go limp.

- Take a warm bath or shower and wash your hair. Feeling clean often makes fatigue more bearable.

Diet

General Information

When you are breastfeeding, do not try to lose weight by dieting. A well-balanced diet and nutritious snacks will not make you gain weight. You may have to change your shopping and eating habits. If time and convenience are important, it is just as easy to eat an apple as it is a doughnut. You will need to drink at least three quarts of liquid each day (twelve full glasses). There is no set diet or prescribed type of liquids for a breastfeeding mother. Lactation itself is independent of diet. An adequate diet and liquid intake, however, will improve the quality of your milk, make you feel better, and help you regain your strength. This, in turn, makes breast-feeding more successful.

- Eliminate junk foods from your diet but do not become anxious about enjoying an occasional piece of pie or some pretzels; they will not ruin your milk production.

- Select foods that are not likely to affect your babies. Most foods should not present any problems. The majority of foods do not go through to your milk, however, strong spices may. Allergens will, so watch for allergic reactions in your babies (rashes, irritability, etc.).

- Plan your meals around the basics: meat, vegetables, fruit, and cereal products. Keep fruit, cheeses, and unsalted nuts on hand for snacks.

- Consult your doctor before taking any vitamin supplements. Sensible eating may mean you do not need them.

- Do not worry about the need to drink large quantities of milk. Other foods contain the needed calcium. Cow's milk does not help make human milk.

- Pay attention to your thirst. Remember to drink a glass of water as you pass the kitchen or bathroom. Have a glass of juice or milk with you when you sit down to breast-feed. Do not count cups of coffee as part of your required liquids, as caffeine tends to be a diuretic and actually reduces the liquids in your body. Let your thirst determine the amount of liquids you require.

● Use alcohol with common sense. A little will not hurt, but alcohol does go through to your milk. A glass of wine or sherry before breastfeeding may help your relax. Beer or stout may increase your milk at feeding time and these drinks do contain some nourishment, paritcularly the B. vitamins. They aslo help your relax.

● Stop smoking. At the very least, cut down on the number of cigarettes smoked during the day. DO NOT SMOKE WHILE YOU ARE FEEDING THE BABIES.

Breast Care

General Information

You must be extra careful about the care of your breasts while nursing.

Suggestions

● Buy several good nursing brassieres. Wear a clean one every day.

- Use clean handkerchiefs or new diapers cut in squares as breast pads to collect any leakage.

- Take a sponge bath and wash your breasts daily if time does not allow for a shower or full bath.

- Wash off any antiseptic cream before feeding. You do not have to wash your breasts at each feeding if they and your clothes are clean.

- When traveling in hot weather or when a daily sponge-off is not possible, carry a damp washcloth in a plastic bag. Avoid commercial cleaning wipes as they contain alcohol and perfumes that may dry or irritate your nipples.

- Change breast pads frequently if you are having a problem with leakage. If the milk has dried and the pad is stuck, do not pull it away. Moisten it with water on your fingers and gently remove it.

- Avoid using plastic-backed breast pads or plastic-lined nursing bras for prolonged periods of time. The moisture cannot evaporate and may cause nipple skin to break down, increasing any soreness.

9

THE MOTHER OF MULTIPLES AND HER FAMILY

It is important to know about the adjustments that may be necessary in your family before and after the birth of your multiples. The situations mentioned arise because there is more than one baby to care for, not necessarily because you are breastfeeding. If all members of your family are aware of family changes that come along with a multiple birth (i.e., that you will need added support and rest), your breastfeeding experience will get off to a better start.

Rearing two or more infants of the same age is an exciting challenge for parents. Life, at first, may be alternately delightful and difficult, uplifting and frustrating for you and your family. As each child's special personality emerges and develops, the relationships you develop with your babies becomes more positive and fulfilling—a multiple love experience.

Pregnancy and Birth

A multiple pregnancy usually places more physical demands on the mother than does a single pregnancy. Many women experience greater weight gain and fluid retention, abdominal and back discomfort, and increased fatigue due to the activity of two or three infants. If you have other children, meeting daily demands may be very taxing.

Despite the new, sophisticated equipment available to aid in diagnosis of a multiple pregnancy, approximately 40 percent of parents are unaware that they will have more than one baby until delivery. Even with triplets or quadruplets, the diagnosis is often made late in pregnancy or is wrongly assessed as twins. Feelings of panic and shock are common. It is normal to be anxious about possible complications in delivery, to question your ability to cope with two or more babies, to be concerned about the reaction of your older children, and to have financial concerns. Emotional adjustments and mutual support by both parents are necessary at this time.

Hormonal changes, fatigue, and anxiety after birth may make you irritable and discouraged. You may cry for no apparent reason. This period of "blues" may occur while you are still in the hospital, last a day or two, or may persist for several weeks. Mothers of multiples tend to be very excited during the days immediately following their babies' birth and often do not experience these feelings of depression until several weeks after they are home. Many women, of course, never feel this sense of anxiety. Each person's situation will be unique. If you have to leave one or more babies in the hospital, a feeling of depression accompanied by a sense of unreality is very normal.

A major cause for anxiety with mothers of multiples is the feeling that they will not be able to "bond" with more than one baby. Bonding is defined as "uniting or tying yourself in a close relationship." In simple terms, this means the warm maternal feelings you have toward your children. The difficulties you may have experienced during your pregnancy, along with labor and delivery, may delay this sense of bonding. If your expected "one baby" turns out to be more, it is quite normal to have ambivalent feelings about the situation and perceive any additional babies as intruders. You and your whole family need time to adjust to a totally unexpected event. The best method for accomplishing that is to talk about your feelings—not to suppress them.

Prematurity in multiple births is very common and can delay the bonding if the babies must be placed in an intensive care nursery. It is essential that you see and touch your babies as soon as possible after delivery and as often as practical during those early days. It is not unusual for a mother of premature or tiny multiples to feel detached from them. Some mothers express this as "seeming to be an interested observer instead of the mother." This feeling is reduced a great deal if you collect your milk for your babies, thus giving you an active role in their care.

Your husband needs frequent contact with your babies, for he, too, may be shocked and panicked by the event. Not being in the hospital with them really makes him feel like an outsider. Try to schedule talks with your doctor about the babies' health at a time when your husband can be present. Encourage him to read any available literature on multiples.

Family Adjustments Once You Are Home

If you are a first-time mother, you may be feeling unsure of your abilities; mothering is a totally new experience and caring for babies is a 24-hour responsibility. The time consumed in caring for your new babies may make you feel somewhat resentful and socially deprived, especially if you were an active working woman. If you have older children, you may have ambivalent feelings as you again begin the total care of infants while coping with adjustments for your other children. As you gain more experience caring for the babies, your confidence will grow and your feelings of self-doubt or resentment should fade away.

It is not easy to meet the physical and emotional needs of your babies and those of all the other members of your family. Some days you will go to bed feeling that if one more demand is made on you, you will scream or pack up and leave! It is usually about that time that your husband indicates that a quick goodnight kiss is not what he had in mind. Both of you need sexual release and a return to the warmth and joy of truly "making love." In time this will happen, and if you can satisfy your physical needs in whatever moments you can grab together, you will keep your sexual relationship "simmering" until your life returns to a more normal schedule.

If there is any possible way you can have regular help during the first two to three months, get it. This can range from a full-time, live-in nanny to a teenager who comes for two hours after school each weekday. In most Canadian provinces and some states in the U.S.A., there are homemaker services available for short- or long-term help. Since this service comes under a variety of agencies, ask your doctor or the hospital social worker for assistance.

Have your husband or the nursing staff contact your local Parents/Mothers of Twins Club (such groups also welcome parents of triplets or quadruplets). They will have a mother visit you with literature and some helpful advice. Once you are at home, make an effort to get out

to their meetings. You will find sympa-
thy for the bad days and a lot of shared
laughter and joy.

A Note for Fathers

General Information

A multiple birth can bring dramatic
changes in your lifestyle. This is especially true if you are a first-time father.
You will soon become involved in your
babies' world. Your attitude toward baby

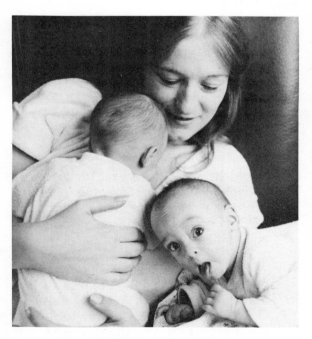

A Double Love Experience

care and breastfeeding will play a big part in how the whole family adjusts. You have the burden of financial responsibility. A reluctance to spend the whole day on a job and then to come home to more work is understandable. You must realize that the time and effort you put into helping with household chores and assisting in the care of the babies is going to bring about a closer relationship with your wife and with your new children.

Suggestions

- Read the books your wife has selected on breastfeeding and infant care.

- Accompany her at least once to visit the doctor before the babies are born and be with her when she consults a pediatrician.

- Begin taking over a greater share of household tasks before the children are born so your wife can rest. These new habits will carry on after the babies are born.

- Assume more responsibility with your older children. Make bath and bedtime your job. Most mothers find the hours from 5 p.m. to 8 p.m. the hardest to get through and will really appreciate time to relax.

- Take a good look at your home and your daily routine and suggest renovations or changes that will save time and steps.

- Be cheerful and accepting in the face of chaos and clutter. The situation will not last forever and your wife cannot relax if she is constantly worried about how you feel about an untidy home or late meals.

- Be patient, please! A multiple pregnancy has probably meant an interruption in your normal sexual activity. Now that the babies are born, your wife goes to bed to sleep...period! This, too, will not last forever. Many couples experience a certain degree of strain in their marriage after a multiple birth. This is not only due to lack of sexual activity caused by exhaustion; your wife may be tense and distracted trying to fit so many activities into her day. She may resent the fact that you are away from "baby care" almost every day. She may be too tired to try to maintain a close relationship with one more person that day. You may feel the strain, perhaps, of an added financial burden. You may resent the fact that your wife now appears not to listen or care about your concerns, or you may miss a lifestyle where you could both come and go at will. Under all this pressure, it is very easy to forget or fail to recognize that something very wonderful and special has happened to your family. Maintain your sense of humor and ENJOY your babies.

Your Older Children

General Information

When multiples arrive in a family after a first child or other children, you will have extra concerns. These offspring have had your attention for a period of time. Jealousy and resentment are normal and can take many forms, depending on the age of the child: a regression to baby-like behavior, thumb sucking, whining, forgetting toilet training, tantrums, or even physical aggression toward the new arrival is common. An older child may become withdrawn or sullen, deliberately ignoring family rules, or may become disruptive in the classroom or neighborhood. A family with two or more older children may face combinations of all these behaviors. The added closeness between you and the babies when you are breastfeeding may at first add to this jealousy or prolong it. There are several ways you can help reduce the negative reactions of an older child.

- Explain to your older child how you fed and cared for him when he was a baby; show family pictures.

- Answer honestly his questions about breastfeeding and do not hide behind closed doors while feeding.

- Do not neglect normal discipline, but be aware of how short your fuse is when you are tired. Be tolerant.

- Plan activities with him that do not always include the babies. Be careful that his father is not always with him and you with the babies.

- Encourage him to verbalize his feelings toward the babies.

- Use feeding times as a time for quiet conversation with him.

- Do not get caught up in the "super mom" myth. You cannot be all things to all people at this particular time in your life. Caring for new babies is probably the most intensive work you will ever do, and an older child will have to accept the few close and quiet moments that you can give him.

- Do not feel guilty if you cannot spend hours on crafts or take him to a variety of classes or activities.

All these special times will return again once you have established your breastfeeding and baby care routine.

Other Family Members

General Information

Parents or other relatives living nearby can be a blessing or a burden. If they recognize your need to adjust to this time of intense baby care and offer constructive, nonintrusive help, you are truly fortunate. Many mothers report that their relatives start a visit with "If you weren't breastfeeding" and go on to list all the things that would be "better." Many mothers put an end to this simply by saying, "If I weren't breastfeeding, I wouldn't be happy."

Suggestions

- Make everyone aware of times you will be resting or your family's need to be alone together.

- Do not let the excitement of your new babies allow others to shut out your older children.

- Never turn down an offer of help, but make sure that such assistance does not create more work or tension for you.

10

THE BENEFIT OF
EXPERIENCE

No amount of reading can replace the benefit of talking to women who have had the experience of breastfeeding their babies. Every mother invents her own shortcuts or variations in positioning and one of them may be just what you need for your situation.

The Center for Study of Multiple Birth's number one rule for new or expectant mothers of multiples is that you contact your local chapter of a Parents/ Mothers of Twins Club as soon as you know that you are expecting multiples. They will help you obtain literature and equipment and can offer lots of hints for baby care. You may not be able to attend regular meetings of these groups when your babies are newborns, but do keep in touch over the telephone and get out as soon as you can. There is a strong bond between mothers of multiples, and you will feel welcome immediately.

Sources for Information

The following organizations can provide you with general information, practical support, and a list of books you may purchase.

• United States:

National Organization of Mothers of
Twins Clubs, Inc.,
5402 Amberwood Lane
Rockville, Maryland 20853
(301-460-9108)   (referral to local
clubs)

The Center for Study of Multiple
Birth
Suite 463-5
333 East Superior Street
Chicago, Illinois 60611
(312-266-9093)

La Leche League International,
Inc. *
9616 Minneapolis Avenue
Franklin Park, Illinois 60131

• Canada:

Parents of Multiple Births Associations of Canada
283 7th Avenue South
Lethbridge, Alberta T1J 1H6
(403-328-9165)   (referral to local
clubs)

La Leche League in Canada
Box 39, Williamsburg
Ontario KOC 2HO

* Check your telephone directory
  for a local chapter.

- Australia:

  Australian Multiple Birth Association
  P.O. Box 151
  Panania, 2213
  N.S.W.   (referral to local clubs)

- Great Britain:

  Twins Clubs Association of Great Britain
  Judi Linney
  198 Woodham Lane, New Haw
  Weybridge, Surrey
  England   (referral to local clubs)

Reading and Reference

Breastfeeding:

- Brewster, Patricia Dorothy, You Can Breastfeed Your Baby Even In Special Situations, Rodale Press, Emmaus, PA, 1979.

- Gromada, Karen K., "Mothering Multiples," La Leche League International, Publication #52, Franklin Park, IL, 1981.

- Health and Welfare Canada, "Breastfeeding: An Awareness Program," (an information kit),

Nutrition Education Unit, Health and Welfare Canada, Ottawa, Ontario, K1A 1B4.

- Health Education Associates, various leaflets on aspects of breastfeeding, 520 School House Lane, Willow Grove, PA, 19090.

- "Helpful Hints for Breastfeeding Multiples," National Organization of Mothers of Twins Clubs, Inc., Rockville, MD, 1981.

- La Leche League International, "The Womanly Art of Breastfeeding, Revised, Franklin Park, IL, 1981.

- Pryor, Karen, Nursing Your Baby, Pocket Books, Harper and Row, NY, NY, 1973.

- Stanway, Penny, M.D, and Stanway, Andrew, M.D., Breast is Best, Pan Books, London, 1978.

- Thorner, Prue, The Simplicity of Breastfeeding, New English Pocket Edition, London, 1974.

Twins and Triplets:

- Noble, Elizabeth, Having Twins: A Parent's Guide to Pregnancy, Birth and Early Childhood, Houghton Mifflin, Boston, MA, 1980. (Available from the Center for Study of Multiple Birth and POMBA).

- POMBA, "Special Delivery [3]," a booklet for parents of triplets. (Available from the Center for Study of Multiple Birth and POMBA.)

- Theroux, Rosemary, R.N., and Tingley, Josephine, R.N., <u>The Care of Twin Children: A Common-Sense Guide for Parents</u>, The Center for the Study of Multiple Birth, Chicago, IL., 1978. (Available from the Center in for Study of Multiple Birth and POMBA.)

<u>Quadruplets:</u>

- POMBA, "Coping with Quads," (Available from the Center of Study of Multiple Birth and POMBA).

BOOK LISTS AND OTHER INFORMATION ARE AVAILABLE FROM:

- The Center of Study of Multiple Birth, free. Enclose a self-addressed, stamped envelope.

- POMBA - $1.00. Published each August, and subject to availability.

- NOMOTC's "Your Twins and You." free. Enclose a self-addressed, stamped envelope.

THE ONE STOP TWIN BOOK SHOP

The Care of Twin Children: A Common Sense Guide for Parents, by Theroux and Tingley (7th printing). "The best twin care book now available," Kay Mossell, *The New York Times*. If you only buy one book on twin care, choose this one! Illustrated, 1978, 120 pp. **Single Copy: $6.75; 2 to 10 copies: $6.50 ea; 11 to 20 copies: $5.95 ea; 21 to 50 copies: $5.50 ea; Library Edition: $14.95 ea.**

Breastfeeding Twins, Triplets and Quadruplets: 195 Practical Hints for Success A guide for mothers who want to breastfeed twins, triplets or quadruplets. Illustrated, 1982, 100 pp. **$4.95 ea.**

Twins: Nature's Amazing Mystery, by Kay Cassill. Written by a twin, it has 320 pages in a hardcover, 5-5/8" × 8-1/2" book. Packed with arresting information, this book is the first of its kind to examine, in a cultural, historical, and scientific context, the extraordinary phenomenon of multiple births. **Single copy: $16.00; 2 to 10 copies: $15.40 ea; 11 to 20 copies: $14.25 ea; 21 to 50 copies: $13.25 ea.** (Includes $1.05 postage and handling)

Twins on Twins, by Kathryn McLaughlin Abbe and Frances McLaughlin Gill, the foremost female photographers in the U.S. They capture the fascination and mystery of twins and twinship with over 100 exquisite photos and thoroughly researched text. 9" × 12". **Single copy: $19.75; 2 to 10 copies: $19.05 ea; 11 to 20 copies: $18.30 ea; 21 to 50 copies: $17.80 ea.** (Includes $1.80 postage and handling per copy)

Having Twins, by Elizabeth Noble. This book focuses on the period from conception through the first few weeks of life. A *must* for women who have an early diagnosis of twins. **$9.25 ea.** (Includes $1.30 postage and handling)

The Triplets. Mattie, Patty and Hattie were triplets. All three of them looked and dressed alike. How Mother, Father, Miss Vigger, their teacher, and Robert Peabody, a classmate, think up a plan to tell them apart makes an amusing and satisfying climax to a story about individuality that will be appreciated by triplets and non-triplets alike. A picture book. 32 pp. 9" × 9". **$7.95 ea.**

Poems About Twins compiled by the Fort Worth MOTC. This is a rare collection of poems about twins written by many parents. **Single copy: $2.50; 2 or more copies: $2.25 ea.**

Special Delivery 3, Triplets. Written by Canadian parents of triplets. A help for new parents of "Supertwins," it incorporates thoughts and suggestions of many families willing to share their experience. **$1.50 ea.**

Two of Everything But Me, by Marion B. West. Marion is a mother of twins who writes about the agony and ecstacy of multiple birth parenting with candor and humor. **Single copy: $3.95; 2 or more copies: $3.75 ea.**

TERMS AND CONDITIONS

- Orders shipped within 7 days.
- All purchases are unconditionally quaranteed at the time of delivery and for 10 days thereafter.
- If you are not satisfied for any reason, return the book in **resalable** condition within **10 days** for a full refund. **After this time write for per-mission to return.**
- Prices and availability of books are subject to change without notice. **All prices quoted are in U.S. dollars.** Out-of-stock titles will be back-ordered.

ORDERING INSTRUCTIONS

1. List book title in spaces provided.
2. Complete the shipping information on the form.
3. Include the correct postage and handling.
4. Attach this form to your check.

5. Send this completed form with remittance (check) to:
   Center for Study of Multiple Birth
   Suite 463-5, 333 E. Superior Street
   Chicago, Illinois 60611   **(312) 266-9093**

PREPAID ORDERS ONLY (U.S. Funds Only)

Title	Price	No. Copies	Amount
	Subtotal		
	Postage and Handling **$1.00** on all orders less than **$6.75**		
	Grand Total		

Name _____

Club _____

Address _____

City _____

State _____ Zip _____

TERMS AND CONDITIONS

- Orders shipped within 7 days.
- All purchases are unconditionally guaranteed at the time of delivery and for **10 days** thereafter.
- If you are not satisfied for any reason, return the book in **resalable** condition within **10 days** for a full refund. **After this time write for permission to return.**
- Prices and availability of books are subject to change without notice. **All prices quoted are in U.S. dollars.** Out-of-stock titles will be back-ordered.

ORDERING INSTRUCTIONS

1. List book title in spaces provided.
2. Complete the shipping information on the form.
3. Include the correct postage and handling.
4. Attach this form to your check.

5. Send this completed form with remittance (check) to:
   Center for Study of Multiple Birth
   Suite 463-5, 333 E. Superior Street
   Chicago, Illinois 60611   (312) 266-9093

PREPAID ORDERS ONLY (U.S. Funds Only)

Title	Price	No. Copies	Amount
		Subtotal	
		Postage and Handling $1.00 on all orders less than $6.75	
		Grand Total	

Name _____

Club _____

Address _____

City _____

State _____ Zip _____